When times get tough and it seems like you can't do it anymore, take some time and reflect on *who* **they** are in your life.

When the day is long and your patience is short, reflect on *why* you are giving your all.

When you feel unappreciated and wonder if your efforts make a difference, know *what* you do matters!

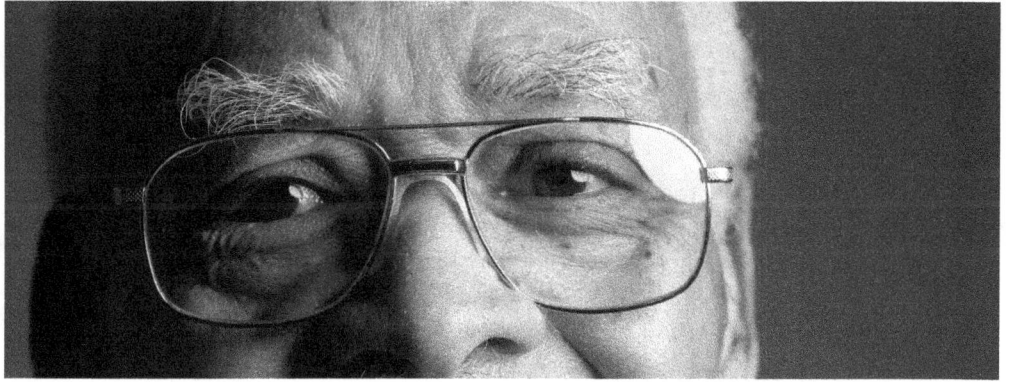

DAD'S GOT DEMENTIA

...

LIFE AFTER DIAGNOSIS

BY
SHELLEY CHATMON HALL

ISBN: 978-0-9995694-0-5 [print]

Manufactured in the United States of America

To My Dad, William T. Chatmon, Sr.

I've written this book in honor of you, dad, after you were diagnosed with vascular dementia in 2010 (currently still living with this disease). I know you would be proud that I am trying to help others. You set the example for us by how you lived your life – always willing to help someone else with encouraging words, being there for them and lending financial support.

Thank you ...

Mom, for providing a safe, clean and loving environment for my father to be cared for and nurtured at home in his familiar surroundings. For the many hours you have spent preparing home cooked meals for him and altering your menu's when his dietary needs change. You too, are so strong and I appreciate you.

My eldest brother, William T. Chatmon, Jr. (Tommy) who sacrifices every single day by making dad's life your career. You are dad's full-time caregiver and unselfishly care for his every need. You give so much of yourself and your time. Your wife, Tonya, has to be equally admired for standing behind you and encouraging you on. Words can't express how much you both are valued.

My other siblings, Pam, Melodie and Kevin. You have cared for dad and continue to sacrifice your time to help him enjoy his life. Giving your own special gifts to keep dad amused, fed, encouraged and loved.

My loving husband, Curtis Hall. You pushed me to etch my thoughts on paper to share with others. I doubted being able to do it and even asked for a ghost-writer. I am thankful for many things. One is how you always encourage me and another is how you treat my dad as your own by being right in the trenches with all of us in his daily care.

Contents

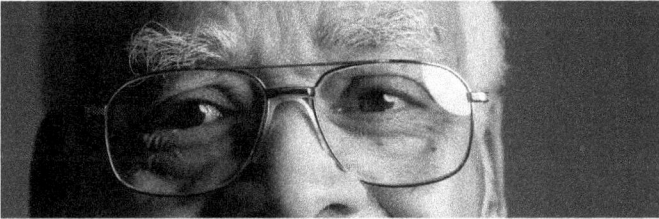

CHAPTER ONE

THE BIG "D"

THERE WERE THREE life-changing moments that led to Dad being diagnosed with vascular dementia. Many of us have heard phrases like, "Your life can change in an instant" or "In a blink of an eye." Well, that had little meaning to me prior to the three events that changed the trajectory of our entire family's future. Our lives changed the moment we heard those words, "vascular dementia."

Wait ... what? What does that mean? Should we be afraid? Is he going to die? Can you fix it?

After the initial shock of hearing those words, and it sinking in a bit, I had to step back and ask, "What in the world is vascular dementia anyway?"

Due to dad's high blood pressure, the doctor indicated that it was caused by mini strokes that, in most instances, go undetected. Okay, so it's caused by mini strokes as a result (in most cases) of high blood pressure. So all we need to do is make sure we keep his blood pressure under control and avoid those mini strokes from happening. Right?

As we would soon find out, controlling blood pressure wasn't even the half of it! And it wasn't the solution to "fixing" this dementia thing.

Back to those three life-changing moments – those dreadful events that led to Dad's diagnosis and our emotional roller coaster: The first happened one Saturday morning. My mom, sister and Dad decided to go out of town to attend a family baby shower. It was a beautiful day for a drive, and the destination was only two hours away. However, minutes into the drive, my father realized it was Saturday, the day that we normally attended church and the time scheduled for him to participate in our communion service. You are probably wondering why that would that be life-changing?

You have to understand that my dad was a very spiritual man. He was dedicated to the church and the obligations he had there. He *never* missed communion. *NEVER EVER!* He expressed confusion over how or why he could have forgotten something that was engrained in him – something so important to him. He went back home, dressed for church and stayed true to his commitment.

The second event happened another Saturday, very shortly after the first one. We were at my parents' house for Saturday dinner. My dad said that at church he had stood from a kneeling praying position and had fallen backwards into the pew. His head had fallen back and he had lost control of his body for a few seconds. That obviously scared him because otherwise he would not have told us about it. We were all very concerned, but my sister Melodie was the one who took action. She insisted that he needed to make a doctor's appointment to get checked out. When he didn't do it, she made the doctor's appointment that would eventually give us the words no one wants to hear.

Before the diagnosis, but during the same month as the first two life-changing events, my mother confided in me that notices from the bank were coming to the house and she didn't know what to do about them. She said she asked my dad about the notices that read "Foreclosure," but he said not to worry – that he would take care of it.

At first she didn't worry, but every day more and more notices arrived, with the threat of severe consequences. She was terrified of what was happening but not sure how she should handle it.

So you better understand her confusion, this was outside of her role in our family. Growing up, our family dynamics were very traditional and remained long after my siblings and I were all grown and out of the house. When we would come over every weekend, the traditional interactions remained. My dad took total care and responsibility of my mom, her needs, their life and their finances. You name it, and he did it! She never really concerned herself with her own survival or existence. She chose to work a part-time job, and her money was her mad money. That was the life! Not a care in the world about her living expenses.

Dad was from the era in which men were totally responsible for their wives and families, unlike today, where the roles are sometimes reversed or shared. That arrangement worked for them – until it didn't. And that's when we were pulled in.

I took the notices Mom provided and talked to Dad about them. Of course, when I stepped in to help, the mortgage was already pretty far into delinquency, and I needed to scramble to gather information in order to help. I noticed that physically Dad appeared quite relieved to have me take over this responsibility. It was as if a heavy burden had been taken off his shoulders. He willingly and possibly even gladly relinquished all financial obligations and turned the management of his finances over to me.

In a matter of four weeks' time, we had gone from a fun-loving family to a family in full panic mode. With not all of us totally on board or accepting of what changes were coming – All hands on deck!

All three life-changing moments happened during these four weeks. We were able to quickly put the pieces together and make (some) sense of what was happening. While we didn't have all the answers, my siblings and I were smart enough to know that we had to step in and put a plan in motion to resolve the situations we could and strategize for the future on the others.

That day at the doctor's office was the first day of a changed life for us and for my dad. But what did it all mean? The doctor diagnosed him with "vascular dementia." She prescribed a drug called *Namenda* and instructed him to take it every single day to slow the pace of his memory loss. We gratefully took the prescription and hopefully prayed we had caught it in enough time to stop whatever it was that was coming. I felt if he missed one dosage that one more small piece of his memory was gone, never to be retrieved. For a while, I secretly believed that this small pill would allow us to continue as usual with dad fixing dinners, laughing and joking and just remaining the strong head of our family.

Before Dad was formally diagnosed with vascular dementia in the early spring of 2010, he was a very social man – not just with family but with friends and strangers alike. We spent many weekends together as a family – as grown kids with our own kids. Saturday family dinners kept us all connected – five kids, spouses and grandchildren filled Mom and Dad's house with lots of noise, unruly outbursts, uncontrollable laughter, exaggerated storytelling, pranks and constant kitchen/refrigerator runs. My dad loved us all being there. I would later read in one of his journals that it made him very happy to have us all home.

Most of us can't comprehend that any disease can cause total confusion yet not show (immediate) signs on one's outward appearance. Dad didn't *look* sick. He still drove himself around, went to the grocery store and socialized with family and friends. We still ate dinner together and laughed and joked. Sure, he forgot things here and there, but if that's all it was, we could handle it.

Turns out, that wasn't all it was. There weren't any follow-up appointments to "fix" anything. We were baffled by the perceived lack of support or care. We had hoped for maybe a magic pill invented by modern science, or at least some follow-up appointments to ... I don't know ... maybe check his blood pressure or something?

We started to realize that it wasn't that doctors didn't care but that there wasn't anything they could do. There was no cure for dementia. We were sent home without plans for the future or expectations of anything other than short-term memory loss for him and somewhere down the road, long-term memory loss. But still, what did that really mean? How can there not be a follow-up to "fix" this?

Look, I work in corporate America. It's my job, your job, our jobs to come up with solutions for some simple and some complex problems. Problem solving is a part of a skill set I'm expected to have to be successful and meet my client expectations. I can truly pat myself on the back. Problem solving has always been one of my strongest skills so you can imagine my initial feelings and thoughts towards the doctors. It went something like this (in my mind), "You're a doctor and much smarter than I am! I mean, I have a Master degree in business but you, you went to medical school and had to learn all the body parts, blood, nerves, joints, tendons, and all that other stuff. I don't understand why you aren't able to solve this problem? If there is an issue, just solve it!"

Yep! I wasn't thinking so clearly. This was the very first medical crisis in our immediate family. Initially, we were at a real loss as to what to do; however, instinct for family survival kicked in, and we moved swiftly. And if you're experiencing a similar crisis, you should move swiftly too.

Part of your survival strategy is reading this book to at least get you started down the journey of providing the best care and comfort possible. I would love to tell you that this book will give you a step-by-step guide to surviving the recent diagnosis of dementia. Every 66 seconds someone develops dementia and the fact is that it's a complicated situation to navigate, and every experience can be unique.

This book is intended to give you some information to think about and share with your family. It will get you started and help you develop a plan of your own for other situations that will need to be addressed as you care for and make decisions for your loved one. It will show you that life isn't over after the diagnosis. It's just different.

CHAPTER TWO

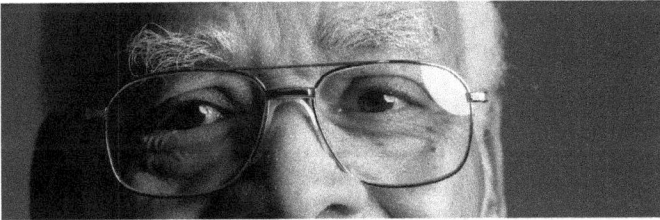

EDUCATE YOURSELF, FAMILY, FRIENDS AND LOVED ONE

A NY TYPE OF HEALTH CRISIS is difficult to wrap one's mind around. The initial shock can set even the best of us back and paralyze us with fear. It may even cause some denial on your part. I know my reaction to most things is to think of the absolute worst that can happen and plan from that point. That strategy might not work for everyone. That is how I cope with any type of problem, and that is how *I* imagined my siblings and I would handle our current health crisis.

I failed to factor in that none of us even knew what vascular dementia really was. We had a pre-conceived notion from the doctor's visit that it was caused by mini strokes and, if these were controlled, that would then stave off further mental decline. That theory was soon checked off as "INVALID" the first time my father's symptoms became a bit more evident.

Our first plan of attack was to move my parents closer to our side of town, so we could help them if we needed to. We didn't understand the true impact a mind-altering disease, such as dementia, could have on someone's ability to carry out such simple daily tasks like bathing, eating or communicating a need. So "helping" was truly an understatement, though we didn't realize it at the time.

While house hunting for my parents, we walked into a house that was just perfect for them. As we walked through, I remember my father making a joke and having a child-like grin on his face after he'd told it. I laughed nervously because I didn't know where "that look" came from. Envision this if you will. My dad stands 6'5 ½ tall, weighs 225 pounds, wears a size 16 ½ shoe and has super-sized hands. He doesn't look (or sound) like a wimpy weakling! Nor was he one.

Dad was always a strong, towering figure that could command anyone's attention when he walked into a room. Handsome, strong and full of vitality, charisma and spunk. Where does a child-like grin ever fit into a persona such as his? I hadn't seen it before, and I found it disturbing and perplexing. How could I process what I just saw?

After several more small but significant incidents, I knew this was something we needed to investigate fully. Short-term memory loss meant more than just forgetting to close the door. I was beginning to understand just how memory loss could manifest itself.

After we decided on a new house that was closer to us, my parents settled into it nicely. It was a ranch-style home, with a fenced-in perfectly landscaped back yard on a cul-de-sac and in a quiet neighborhood with other mature adults. They loved the tranquility and natural beauty of it all.

One afternoon, mom called me in a panic! They (mom and dad) were on their back porch, she had gone into the house for only a second to get some water. When she came out, dad was laying on the ground on his back with the full afternoon sun beating down on him. At first glance, she thought he was dead. Once she reached him, she realized he was alive, but he couldn't get up and she couldn't get him up. My husband and I live within minutes so we were like super-hero's moving faster than the speed of light getting there. And, I'm pretty sure we weren't following the rules of the road because we were riding on two wheels around those corners.

Our guess is that dad must have gotten up from the swing they were sitting on. Maybe he tried to sit back down and missed the swing landing on the ground. Thankfully, he didn't get hurt!

Strange part was that he could have easily sat and then stood up by himself. The swing was right behind him and he could have used it to help himself get up. But he didn't. He didn't know how to get up. He could not get off of his back into a standing position because his brain couldn't comprehend those complex maneuvers; arms, legs, feet, move, push, pull... Strange right? On top of all of that, he never even tried to shield his face from the sun. Now do you see what I mean about our theory being "Invalid"?

Given these newer developments, my sisters and I committed ourselves to researching this mind-altering disease called dementia. Or was it Alzheimer's or vascular dementia? Those names were often used interchangeably, and we weren't really sure if there were differences. We all read everything we could find on the internet about dementia. Some seemed like credible information, some not so much (offering that "magic pill" to cure all or eating 10 eggs in one sitting). But we just needed to know everything!

During our research we learned that the types (Vascular, Alzheimer's, Lewy body, etc.) tree up to dementia. I recently heard a great explanation of dementia that is easy to understand. Let's say you've been diagnosed with cancer so the type could be melanoma or breast cancer. Same for dementia. You've been diagnosed with dementia and the type is Alzheimer's, Vascular or Lewy Body. Get it?

To further complicate things, in researching the topic you will quickly run into the "stages" of this disease. The different stages are: 1 – 7; mild, moderate and severe; or early, mid and late stages. Each stage is represented by a description of behaviors at that point and what it will be at the next stage. It is sort of a tracker to let you know what to expect and when that person is in the final stages. Over time, the individual's communication skills will decline. Their ability to problem-solve will diminish. The ability to manage financial obligations will be nonexistent. Managing personal care will be impossible for them; as will, feeding oneself, dressing oneself and the list goes on.

I think I can tell you what this information will do to you. You will read the "stages," and try to pinpoint the exact "stage" of the behaviors your loved one is exhibiting. After all, we all have a need to know, and you should know as much as you can to be armed to provide care. However, I need to caution you, even though I already know it won't kick in right away.

It is likely that you and your family will become obsessed with these stages. The first time you hear your loved one utter a jumbled sentence or see them misuse their fork, you are going to run to the list to see how close to that last stage they are. You will continue to do this and will notice that behaviors appear as severe one day and moderate the next day. Please consider that these stages should be used only as an approximate guide to understand the general progression of the disease. They are not exact. Every individual is different, but each will fluctuate many times through the stages. Do not be alarmed!

I have found this chart can be discouraging and cause family members too much anxiety. Let me help put this in perspective for you. The list does not provide any tips on providing care. It will not add to the health or happiness of you or your family. While it's somewhat helpful information to know, when you find yourself becoming obsessed, it's time to leave the list alone and just enjoy your time together, regardless of the "stage."

I recommend that you locate credible sources that will give you a good overview of what dementia is. Start by asking your primary care physician for information on elder care and dementia. They should be able to refer you to the appropriate resources in your area. It is also a good idea to have a geriatric physician involved with their care if they are elderly. Include your siblings, the grandchildren, the one suffering from dementia, family and close friends. It is very important that you help educate each other and those that will be providing some level of care along this journey.

It's also a good idea to gently inform your loved one about their condition so they are on-board for some of the legal concerns that will need to be addressed. Don't become frustrated if you have to explain things multiple times. Don't be surprised if they don't believe you. It's not important to drill it into them. They are probably experiencing short-term memory challenges and won't remember what you shared with them earlier. Just lovingly reassure them that everything will be all right – that you will be there for them. And repeat information whenever necessary.

It is super-duper important to start the education and knowledge-sharing process together as a family – siblings, husbands, wives and grandchildren. This is too big a journey to go alone. You will need all the emotional support you can get – especially in the early stages of the disease after it is diagnosed.

I remember being consumed and overwhelmed with all the information I found online. I needed help sifting through the sites, editorials, personal testimonials and on and on. To help you avoid this initial information overload, I've tried to summarize information for you here. It can all be shocking and scary, but it doesn't have to be that way.

Gather a few credible brochures from Alzheimer's Association, sit down together and go through them. Ask each other questions, share your feelings on what you are reading and just try to absorb it. Have frequent open dialogue as you learn more and begin to realize the diagnosis is real. It helps!

Once my dad was hospitalized during the mid stage of dementia. He was still able to understand many things although he was noticeably impaired. My sisters and brothers and I stayed around the clock with dad at the hospital and at one point, the girls each took turns being the cry baby. If you started with one tear rolling down your cheek, you were politely ushered out of the room by the other two. It actually became funny if you were the one being pushed out.

Shielding dad from our emotional outburst was the goal. That is why I don't recommend including your loved one in the initial investigative phase which we were still in at that time. There are too many emotions the family will have to process, and your emotions can be difficult to control. Besides, you want to be able to speak freely about what you are learning without having to be sensitive to your mom, dad or spouse sitting there. They will need your emotional support and assurance that everything is going to be okay. This is not a time for them to see how uneasy and scared you really are. They already know something isn't right with them. They need to be continually affirmed that the family is there for them and will protect them and stick with them through the changes that are happening.

A few months after diagnosis, we took my dad to his doctor's appointment. He had a great visit and as we stood in the lobby, myself and my mother needed to use the restroom. I walked away, my mother had just begun to walk away and my larger-than-life father said to her, "please don't leave me alone." Talk about heart-breaking! I tear up every time that particular memory comes up. Of course now we reassure my dad through the tone of our voice, physical touch and eye contact and we do not leave him alone. Sometimes he gets sick of us looking at him square in his eyes or touching all on him. We keep it up though! He can't get rid of us girls!

As you share information together and what that means for you as a family, be sure that each of you commit to not being the "weak link" in the group. What do I mean by that? So glad you asked.

Being the "weak link" simply means failing to support other members of your support system through this entire process. I hate to break it to you, but this is going to be a long journey for most.

If you have family conflicts, it's time to resolve them. It will be a very difficult journey if only one family member is on board and providing care and everyone else is disgruntled. Being the caregiver can be physically and emotionally exhausting, with no time to spare on those extra feelings and emotions from *other* family issues. Family differences will only hurt everyone involved. That isn't the type of environment you want for your family member at this point in their life, is it? Pull together! Now is the time! Lean on each other. Confide in each other. Divulge your fears and frustrations ... constructively. You will be surprised that other family members are likely feeling the same things you are.

Commit to helping out consistently. Don't leave it on one person to carry the load! If one parent has been diagnosed, the other parent needs help caring for the sufferer. If it is your spouse, reach out to your children or a caregiving agency for support. I know you will want to protect your special person and may even feel a bit ashamed of what is happening. Trust me when I tell you, shielding your loved-one from the families scrutiny may unintentionally subject them to a not so safe environment. There will be late-night hospital runs – dropping everything to run over to help when mom or dad are not being cooperative. (That definitely will come). You will get tired. You will miss some days at work. You will miss that girls' weekend away. You may miss the basketball game. You might gain a few pounds in the process ... ugh! But, this is a commitment fueled by love. There can't be any other motive or the care just won't be sustainable. It *must* be love!

I felt it was really important to include grand-children in this process. Sure, you will have to tailor the message to fit the age and understanding of the child, but they need to be a part of the process. You want the grandchildren involved for a number of reasons. First, children need to understand what "family" means, and this is an invaluable opportunity to learn this lesson. "Family" means a commitment to each other through thick and thin. Family is your ride-or-die! Meaning, if all your friends leave you, family will always be there for you. If this concept hasn't been instilled in them before now, it's not too late. Children need to understand the obligation we all have not just to *our* family elders but also to elders in our communities. If you don't agree, think about it this way: If or when you become stricken with a health issue, will your children, nieces or nephews know how to help you? Or what's worse, will they *want* to help you? If you are not showing them by example and by their own involvement, your youngsters will miss these life lessons, and they will not be there for your generation when needed.

Another reason to involve the grandchildren (baby, toddler, preteen or teen) is because of the apparently unexplainable effect it has on our loved one with dementia. It is therapeutic! Don't believe me? Give it a try!

A few years into the progression of the disease, my father stopped talking. He would say one or two words but really just didn't want to open his mouth and say anything. We tried everything to get a response from him beyond him shaking his head or gesturing with his hands. My mom asked him why he wouldn't talk and he just said he didn't want to.

With this disease, it is likely that *your* loved one will stop communicating at some point in time too. In our family, we push through these challenges and never just let a decline happen without a fight. For example, dad stopped walking at one point. We had to fight through it and keep exercising his legs and supporting him as he stood to strengthen his legs. (That's another story for another time.)

So during dad's nonverbal stage, dad's one year old great-grandson came over one day and, as soon as Dad saw him waddling around, Dad reached out his hands to him, wanting him to come. He said, "Hey boy!" And the chatter was nonstop from there. You should see how Dad's face lights up whenever any child comes around. Sometimes we take him to the park and wheel him around the playground just so he can see children laughing and playing. This reaction is not confined to just my dad. Other families have the same experience when children and young people come around. This is something that seems to snap them out of being withdrawn. It is a wonder to witness!

It's important to keep our loved one engaged as long as possible When the dementia patient is withdrawn from lack of stimulation they may become quiet. They might avoid interacting with others. If allowed, they will sit for long periods of time staring into nothingness. Imagine looking in their eyes and no one looking back at you. You wave your hand in front of their face and ... nothing.

Isolation and lack of engagement in life, further increases the withdrawal, and will lead to them slowly drifting farther and farther away. Engagement keeps them stimulated and their brain active. There is a fine balance however, so be careful not to over stimulate and cause them to become uncomfortable, uncooperative or combative. Too much stimulation can be irritating and get on their nerves. Too much activity can seem fast or loud. Not good!

With all that's required, managing care can be a lonely road. Believe me when I say your mom, dad, spouse or patient's friends will stop coming around after the initial revelation of their friend's condition. It can be uncomfortable for those friends to come by not knowing what to say. Maybe your loved one is regressing and talking about things in their childhood as if it were just yesterday. Maybe they are asking the exact same question over and over as if they've never asked it before. Maybe they are looking at their friends as if they were total strangers. Or maybe they just spewed out words that are unintelligible while waiting patiently for an answer. Talk about awkward! Most people don't know how to handle this type of exchange and it's best not to blame them. Just because you've done your research and know how to go with the flow doesn't mean friends have. This may be new to their friends and a very unfamiliar situation to be in. Relax and just know that your *new* support system is who you can rely on for visiting and companionship. I'm not suggesting you discount these friends. I'm just suggesting you not be alarmed when the only regular knock on the door is the delivery truck dropping off that recurring order of adult diapers.

Since it's now going to be your support system (siblings or other family) involved and present, make the best of it. Believe it or not, these awkward conversations with your loved one can actually be some funny times. Keep your sense of humor. It's okay to laugh! Answer your family member's random unorganized or unintelligible question any way you want to. Most times if you are paying attention to what they are doing or looking at, you can kind of figure out what they are trying to say. Even if you can't figure it out, respond anyway, and they will either agree and carry on, or look at you like *you* have dementia!

As you research, you'll come to understand more about dementia, communicating with and caring for your loved one. As if you need another definition, here's an easy explanation of dementia. It is any brain-altering condition that results in memory loss, whether gradual, rapid or instantaneous. The differences in the types of dementia are the causes and how the disease progresses. Here are just a few types of dementia that you may recognize: Alzheimer's disease, Vascular Dementia, Lewy body dementia, Frontal-temporal dementia, Parkinson's disease – just to name a few. Alzheimer's is the most common and then vascular dementia is second in line (my dad has vascular). Alzheimer's is a brain disease and vascular dementia is blood supply disease (circulatory) both affecting brain function and memory.

I remember thinking that dementia was "just" memory. I don't remember the doctor ever mentioning anything *other* than a loss of memory. But dementia is more than just forgetting things like car keys or groceries. Take a moment to think about what the loss of brain function *really* means. You need your brain to do everything! Your brain controls your body. Your brain tells you when you're hot, cold, hungry, sad, and mad, lift your leg, sit, stand, walk, eat, swallow, bathe, poop, pee, smile, read. I know you are getting the gist of what I am implying.

If your brain is impaired, someone will have to help you move your leg to take a step forward.

Someone will have to let you know you haven't eaten today, or it's time to drink a glass of water to remain hydrated. Someone may be helping you trace the letters of your name on a piece of paper, and you still don't recognize what those things called "letters" are. Someone will have to keep a close eye on you so you don't wander outside in your pajamas, without shoes, hat or coat. Someone needs to be on standby to take that bottle of cleaning solution out of your hands, because you thought it was lotion. Someone will have to tell you that pepper doesn't go on toast but butter does.

Someone will have to speak to you slowly, using short sentences, looking you in the eye while using gestures and demonstrating so you understand. For your loved one with dementia, that "someone" is you, your family and maybe a very close friend.

Do your research and remember that dementia is bigger than just loss of memory. Think bigger and broader regarding what a decline in thinking and reasoning skills really means. You will need that broader understanding as you move forward in this book and develop your own plan of attack!

So, let's get started!

CHAPTER THREE

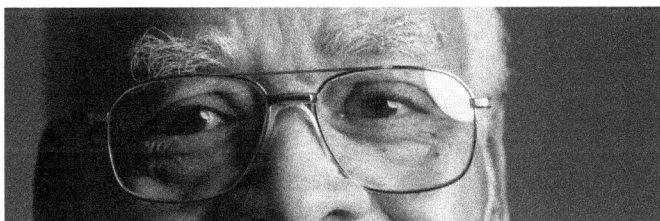

BUSINESS MATTERS

AFTER I HAD SPOKEN to both my mother and father about the threat of foreclosure on their home, I needed to take action to salvage what I could. Not only did I need to resolve the house issue but, more importantly, their financial stability. I worked with an attorney on the house and other financial obligations that were impacted. The good news was that, at that point, Dad was still sufficiently able to understand what was happening. He was able to participate in the discussion by giving approval for people to talk to me, while allowing me to make the decisions. He joined all of the meetings I set up, even though I basically ran the meetings, and he signed all the documents. Taking the lead was just not in his comfort zone any more. He and I were a great team and managed to take care of so many things like that before the first big decline happened. His organized record keeping had not been tampered with so being able to pull documents was easy for him. This saved loads of time!

Being able to manage business matters and not have your name "officially" on contracts and other documents isn't ideal. At the time, I didn't know how much legal control was needed. I remember one day talking to a family friend whose mother was also going through the same mental decline due to dementia (not sure what type). Her mother was a lot farther along than my dad, so at the time she had more experience than we did. I remember one quick tip she gave me – to make sure we got power of attorney for finances and medical care. She had had an experience with going to the doctor, and the doctor not wanting to give her information unless she had that piece of paper.

That was some of the most important advice I could have ever received, so I am imparting it to you. This is a family discussion that needs to be had now. If your loved one is still able to communicate whom they trust with their finances, that person should be assigned POA (Power of Attorney) to help manage finances. One of the most common ways dementia is discovered is through financial negligence. As a result of not being able to manage budgeting and payment schedules, many have lost lots of cash, property and benefits. Short term memory may not even allow them to ask for help.

Handling someone else's money will be sticky at first. The family needs to agree and understand the meaning of a POA. The person with POA has been entrusted to manage the resources to the best of their ability. They don't need to be hassled about it, made to feel guilty or distrusted by other family members. Unless they have given you reason to doubt their ability to manage the funds or have exhibited some poor decision-making, let them be accountable to the immediate family, but give them the autonomy to get things done. Making financial decisions isn't as easy as it sounds. It can put pressure on that person especially if mom or dad have left their affairs in shambles. I think we can all agree that we want our loved ones to be comfortable at this stage in the game. We don't want them to worry about where their next meal is coming from, will their gas or lights be disconnected or will they have a roof over their head. Sometimes decisions have to be made that all may not agree on but if it means the difference between stability and insanity ... I choose stability! Who has time to fight about it? Someone has to be the one to break the tie – so to speak – of what happens next with mom or dad. Continue to work together with your support system with the common goal of wanting what's best.

If you are the one chosen to hold POA, you must be transparent with the family. They have a right to know what is happening and what you are doing with your loved one's money, possessions and care. Always remember that this is not your money! This is your loved one's money and it should be managed better than you manage your own.

Find out what financial obligations currently exist. Ensure that bills are current and if not, contact the creditor, bank, mortgage company and explain your situation and plan for either repayment or otherwise. Send them a copy of the Power of Attorney. Make sure there aren't any additional documents needed by that entity to ensure you are able to speak and act on your loved one's behalf. Whatever else you do, if in the U.S., don't forget to contact the Internal Revenue Service (IRS). They will assign you a Centralized Authorization File (CAF) Number so that you can handle all tax filings needed. You already know the IRS will be relentless if those taxes aren't filed and paid. Uncle Sam wants his money!

Funny story. I contacted a company over my dad's bill that needed to be paid by the insurance company. I told the lady on the phone that my dad has dementia and I'm trying to get more information on the bill so that I can make sure it's submitted to the insurance company. She proceeded to tell me she couldn't talk to me but needed to talk to my father and he needed to give permission for her to talk to me. I reminded her that my dad has dementia and he wouldn't be able to understand her questions. Since she insisted, I put him on the other line. She asked, "Are you Mr. Chatmon?" I said (in the phone on the other end mind you), "dad, say yes." She said, "Do you give me permission to talk to your daughter?" "Dad, say yes." She asked, "what is your daughter's name?' I said, "Dad, Shelley Hall. You have to say Shelley Hall dad."

Hmmm? What just happened here? In total disbelief I realized this was my new normal. Don't be like me. Get the POA as soon as possible.

So we have the money out of the way. What about medical issues? First, it's important to understand what your loved one's wishes are. Do they want to be resuscitated? Do they want to be given every opportunity to bounce back –meaning they do want to be resuscitated? If you throw my book across the room now, I understand. Are you back with me yet?

This "Do Not Resuscitate" (DNR) discussion has been a thorn in my side for the past few years. Every time we go to the emergency room, that's the first thing the staff wants to know. I have been rude about it to the doctors and nurses. I have ignored them and acted like they are not even talking to me. My sisters have given them some words of wisdom like, "If you all ask me that one more time!"

It still doesn't stop them. They are relentless!

When the medical professionals ask, "Does he want to be resuscitated?" what we hear is, "He is an 80-year-old man, so death is imminent. If he holds his breath too long to keep from sneezing, should we just go ahead and pull the plug?"

Our response: "Ma'am, we are here because he is constipated. Can we just get an enema and be on our way?!!" I do crack myself up about our perspective. Hey, if it's not communicated effectively, how are we supposed to know what it really means?! We are not in the medical field and apparently not as smart as we should be about such things.

It was pretty obvious a tutorial was in order to get us past this DNR roadblock. My sister was fortunate enough to have a better discussion with an attending physician who explained what it means to DNR *our* dad. Contrary to popular belief, it does not mean the doctors are looking to harvest his organs and sell them on the black market (HA! Am I the only one that thought that?) For us and our dad, it meant that if he should have a heart attack, beating on his chest or having to crack it open for repair to resuscitate him would be more devastating to him and his medical condition. It would cause more damage to his brain (that by the way is already deteriorating) that could not be repaired and his quality of life would be near zero. Because of the vascular dementia and the progression of his disease, he most likely would have no bounce-back and no recognition of life – existing almost like a vegetable.

DNR may mean something else for your loved one, so I would definitely not allow medical professionals to put a blanket statement out there and have you sign it. You need to consider the sufferers overall health, the quality of life they are living with now and what their wishes are. Over time and as the disease progresses, your views on this may and possibly should change. Our initial responses were an absolute, "Yes, resuscitate!" He wasn't at the stage where, in good conscience, we would put that death sentence on him. (Okay, I admit to still feeling a little unreasonably bitter about that DNR).

As time goes by and physical and mental deterioration occurs, you may need to revisit that decision. Nonetheless, don't feel pressured into signing off. Confer with the primary care physician, specialist or whoever has been caring for your loved one long-term. Their opinions should carry more weight than doctors who are just seeing them for slight sniffles in the emergency room (ER). I'm not taking away from the credibility of ER doctors (because they see it all and do it all) only suggesting taking feedback from the ER back to the doctor managing overall and ongoing care.

In order to make these types of decisions, having a medical POA will help you navigate the care and decision-making for your loved one. When time permits, go with them to all the doctors' appointments and let the staff know who you are. Ask what they will need in terms of documentation for you to act on mom or dads behalf. Make sure your telephone number is listed as the main contact for all things medical. Keep a journal and begin listing all the medications and their dosages. Make a copy of their medical cards, driver's license and any other form of ID. Journal all medical conditions and keep that journal handy so that if an emergency comes up, whoever is closest will be able to quickly grab the journal and provide this information to an attending physician or an EMT (emergency medical technician). This has been a life-saver for us every time the ambulance had to be called or for doctors' appointments in general. The first thing asked is, "what medication is he on". They love it when we just hand them the book while we attend to dad in his time of need (although it's more like us getting in the way of the professionals).

Documentation of conditions and medications is a critical component to helping keep your loved one as healthy as possible. If you have taken on the role of caregiver whether part time or full time, you should not just allow any medications to be prescribed. Each medication has numerous side effects and warnings of drug interactions which can be extremely harmful if not heeded or missed. The urologist may not know that the primary care has prescribed something that shouldn't be taken with medication they are about to prescribe. Documentation and awareness of side effects is especially important because ER visits are likely in your future.

My dad is a veteran. He retired from the U.S Army after 30 years of service. He served his country well and earned all of the medical and financial benefits he now needs and receives. With the privilege of having retiree medical coverage, he also has Medicare. I call it a privilege because so many don't have the expanse of coverage needed to be properly cared for but that's an entirely different conversation about which I have strong opinions.

Dad has two sets of doctors – one for private care and another through the VA (Veteran Affairs). It is important to coordinate care between doctors to make sure that if he goes to one, the other is informed. Different doctors have different best recommendations for different situations, and this can sometimes cause unintentional confusion.

My father went through the early to mid stage where he wasn't eating. He dropped an extreme amount of weight and even fainted once when he tried to stand – all due to lack of nourishment. We had been going back and forth to the VA and was in dire straits. He hadn't eating for weeks, and he was just wasting away. We would sit with him and prod him to just take a bite and another bite until him simply couldn't stomach it. It was pandemonium in our family! He said that he just could not taste the food and if he put it in his mouth, it tasted like cardboard. We didn't know that one's taste buds can be affected by dementia and that foods seasoned with heavier spices are better choices during this time. The VA doctor prescribed an appetite medication called, *Megace (Megestrol)*. Can I just say that drug was a wonder drug (in our case)? Within about three days' time, he was back eating like a horse! Oh, we were feeding him everything his heart desired ... and lots of it! For breakfast he had eggs, grits (we live in the south), turkey bacon, potatoes, toast (with sugar free jam as if that made a difference). Life was grand and all was well – that was until a year into him taking Megace. Dad's other primary care doctor contacted us to tell us that the medication had side effects such as blood clotting and dad needed to be taken off of it.

Okay, Dad had been on this medication without any such side effects. We were not going to relive his skeleton phase and have him go back to not eating again! Sometimes you have to make decisions that *you* feel are best for your loved ones. We decided we could by no means subject him to starvation. We needed more time to weigh the options so we did not take him off the Megace until the prescription ran out a few months later. He was eating so well at that time and we hadn't experienced any other episodes of dad not eating so we decided to take the plunge.

The doctor then prescribed another medication for his appetite. I remember picking it up, scanning the label, not noticing anything related to appetite and asking the pharmacist if this was used for appetite. She said it was typically used for elderly patients in nursing homes who weren't sleeping but since the doctor prescribed it for appetite it might help????? *Ding, ding ding!*

That should have been my queue to dig a bit deeper. I'm usually so inquisitive and ask way too many questions. I never let people tell me things and just accept them if it doesn't sound right to me. This definitely was a time I should have been an irritant and continued to probe and have the pharmacist reach out to his doctor. To this day, I am not sure why I didn't stop there and challenge this prescription.

This happened during a time when we were still not aware that we had the power to question a doctor's orders. We didn't understand that we needed to question every medication, its uses and side effects, and decline the medication if we didn't think it best. I believe most doctors would agree that patient care is a partnership. They can't solve for everything without input from the patient or in this case the family.

So against our better judgment we gave my father just two doses of the medication. Those two doses almost cost him his life! He was rushed to the emergency room after not being able to fully wake him all day. At the hospital he began with labored irregular breathing and then went into a deep sleep which lasted almost a week. He had feeding tubes and oxygen and he just slept. He slept peacefully which allowed us time to process what appeared to doctors as the end. Praise God, we are a praying family and had a praying church family that interceded on my dad's behalf. He woke up after a week of no doctor being able to wake him and with those feeding tubes going into his stomach and wouldn't you know, that offensive DNR order looming!

You have power over what happens to your family member. There are plenty of very good doctors, nurses, caregivers, technicians, but you are the advocate! We have to help our medical professionals provide treatment. This should be a collaborative effort with you having the final word regarding implementing the medication or treatment plan the family has decided on. Ask questions. Don't allow general answers to be provided. Ask to see their chart. You will be surprised at the notes included – things of which you were unaware. Every detail is important to you when caring for your loved one. There isn't any piece of information that is not important. Take charge. You hold the power!

CHAPTER FOUR

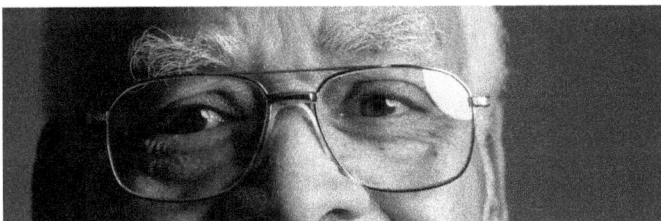

STAGES OF CARE

Y OU ARE ALL FULLY ENGAGED NOW and ready to start planning and executing, right? That's the best place to be in – excited about looking at the situation, accepting the diagnosis and taking it on! I know it's not the kind of excitement you are accustomed to, but trust me, having a plan in place will make things a lot more tolerable. I want to say even enjoyable, even though you might not be ready to hear that yet. It's going to come!

Nothing can be taken for granted when it comes to the everyday living situation of your loved one. My guess is that if you have noticed hints of forgetfulness, confusion, odd language and behavior, then there are many other things happening that you either haven't witnessed yet or have overlooked. That's okay! You understand it now and will pay closer attention. Your family member is depending on the support system that is either already in place or being put in place right now. Take a deep breath! You can do this!

Mom, dad or spouse have probably lived a very independent life up to this point. Many are living in their own homes, apartments or with minimal supervision in an assisted or senior living community. They may drive themselves around to shop or for entertainment and while we certainly want them to have as much independence as possible, safety and care are the primary concerns so it's important to exam where they are in the stage of this disease. With each phase of the disease, their care needs will change. I will caution that you may not agree with my safety views on care, but I am very apprehensive in allowing you to let your guard down at any time during this journey. The unexpected can and will happen when we are not protecting our loved ones and/or patients at every turn. Always keep the thought of a toddler in mind when planning care and supervision. A toddler knows no danger and seems to go for the things that can harm them ... and they're fast! They will reach that "thing" before you realize there even was a "thing".

The moment your loved one was diagnosed, is the moment you should come together with your support system to begin your care plan. It's no longer safe for you to allow your parent, spouse or patient to be in unsupervised conditions. Ponder this. What caused that person to be tested for dementia in the first place? Was it because they were forgetting small things that may have resulted in a larger concern? Was it because they left food on the stove and it caught the kitchen on fire? Was it because they weren't paying their bills and bill collectors were calling?

My dad always managed the bills for the house and continued this practice well after us kids were grown and out of the home. He and mom lived a comfortable life together. He received retirement which was enough for them to live on and still enjoy extracurricular activities. They loved to spend lots of time with the grandkids and take them on short trips, out to dinner or shopping.

Before it was common-place to pay bills online, dad purchased a cashier's check for one thousand dollars to pay his and my mom's mortgage. He lost or misplaced the check and couldn't remember what happened to it. He could not even retrace his steps to the general area where he had been. This was only one of many other times that money mysteriously disappeared without a trace. (Side note), if my husband notices missing money, tell him to check the trunk of my car for those hidden boxes of new shoes first before risking embarrassment and creating *my* care plan! For dad though, it never dawned on us to have him checked out medically.

Although physically dad *looked* perfectly normal and he acted *mostly* normal, he was not normal ... his normal. Had we known or even suspected at that time he could be in trouble, we would have had a jump start on our care plan. We could have avoided more major losses of money, loss of their home, car and insurance policies. Yes, all of these things can and were (eventually) replaced but I'd like to think they could have been avoided. We were blessed that it was only material goods and not he or my mother's safety or loss of life. It isn't that far-fetched to see how it could have been more devastating which is why supervision at this very point in your family member or patient's life is critical. It's important to help them through this new phase of life with a care plan that considers all of the smallest details of their existence.

Let me take a moment to address assisted living, rehabilitation facilities, nursing homes and even hospitals. When you have patients with memory issues it can be difficult to manage. You have multiple patients that each require so much individualized attention. For a time they may look normal just like my dad did. Caregivers may not think as much attention is needed but that is how they may get into trouble. Ways to help avoid falls, wandering or other endangerments is to keep them close or monitoring them often. Incorporate them into activities where you are close by if possible. When visiting a nursing home, I've witnessed a dementia patient at the front desk "helping". I've also witnessed a patient wandering unsupervised and a bit unsteady on their feet. You, as a caregiver, will need the same care tactics that in-home family caregivers use. Our general care plans are the same ... keeping people safe, happy and healthy. You are accountable for the care of your patients. Take pride in how you are caring for and treating them. They will flourish in their new normal because of you.

With the care plan being as important as it is, let's break this down into simple palatable chunks. Complicated isn't going to make it better or easier. Everyone is unique (to a degree) which means that symptoms may vary and daily experiences may differ; however, the general stages we will explore are common and you will gain insight and ideas on how to adapt solutions to fit your unique situation. As we look at stages, we are covering the basic concepts of the level of care needed at each stage of the disease.

Your care plan for each stage of dementia should encompass accommodations, daily support/supervision, physical care, nutrition and exercise. Let's just set the stage by thinking *toddler*! Yes, I said it again – toddler! I understand they are not toddlers and some are offended when using this comparison. For the record, we do not treat dad like a toddler. He won't have it! This reference is the easiest way to begin to think of the type of support that will be needed.

Think back to a time where you either had a toddler of your own or watched someone interact with
their toddler. It's a lot of work but a very fulfilling
experience! It's a good way to begin to think about
the level of supervision and caution needed when
working with the person you will be caring for.

With all stages, having a schedule is pretty
critical to the success of your care strategy. I recommend buying a journal that is kept in the same
location daily. We keep ours in the kitchen cabinet
that also contains doctor's notes, medication, blood
pressure cuff and a few other things. Write the
schedule down so that, as you take turns providing
care with your support team, everyone is on the
same page and knows what must be done.

Each day, date a section of the journal and
write out information that others will need to know
including the doctor. If taking medication, enter
"took all meds". If they refused to take the dosage
or they are out of medicine, annotate that. Did they
eat all of their food for breakfast, lunch or dinner?
Did they pick over their food? Did they have a bowel
movement that day? Are they constipated? Are they
sleeping more often than usual? Are they wandering
during the night? Are they more disoriented today?
Put their daily vitals in the book if you take those
daily. It's really easy to see trends when it's dated
and in black and white.

It may seem like a lot to manage but keep it simple. Date your page and put quick notes in there so the next person caring for your loved one will know to look out for these things. It's also helpful when you can pick the book up and call their doctor and explain how long something has been going on.

If your loved one is in an assisted-living or nursing home, provide a journal so their caregiver can make these same notes. Review the journal each time you visit looking for trends or changes.

Family members, ask the caregiver to provide you with a schedule of the care provided each day. What time are they being awakened, bathed, fed, exercise, offered bathroom breaks, fluid intake, meals, activities, etc? Remember, you are the advocate. If they are unable to provide you with what is being done, how often and when, you might want to take a closer look at the care that's being provided. Exactly what is going on in the daily life of your loved one? Do you know?

If you are a caregiver, make the journaling suggestion to your management team. This will amp up awareness to what is going on with the patient you are caring for. This will also help the next caregiver when your shift is over. You will begin to pay closer attention to improvements or declines in your patient's health or well-being. Further, it will be easier for you to give an update to your patient's family when they call or visit. You can simply pick the journal up and give them an overview of concerns or maybe a funny conversation your patient had with you. Plus, it will help with everyone's accountability and ownership in the patients care.

Our loved ones should be on a schedule very similar to the one below. If you are providing care at home, your schedule should look as detailed as ours below:

First Shift 8:00 — 10:00
Caregiver: William

8:00–9:00	Shower, shave and bathe	Shave — Mon, Wed & Fri.
9:00–10:00	Breakfast	Clean up bathroom, strip and make bed
9:40–10:00	Devotion	

Second Shift 10:00 — 2:00
Caregiver: Sarah

10:00–10:30	Exercise	Walk around house, stand in kitchen with a chore (folding clothes, organizing drawer, reading & opening mail/newspaper). If weather is nice, take outside in wheel chair down to cul-de-sac and to end of street.
10:30–10:50	Bathroom break	Sit on toilet with magazine for 10 minutes, change protective underwear.
11:00–11:30	Cognitive activity	In sitting room or sunroom **without TV**. Puzzle, cards, reading, writing, hold conversation

11:30–12:45	Rest & TV time	Bring back into sitting room and elevate feet. **Provide/offer fresh ice water**
1:00–1:30	Lunch	In kitchen in chair. Put pillow behind upper back and large pillow under his feet so they aren't dangling.
1:30–1:45	Bathroom break	Sit on toilet with magazine for 10 minutes, sponge off with soap and water, and change protective underwear.
1:45–2:00	Rest & TV time	Bring back into sitting room and elevate feet. **Provide/offer fresh ice water.**

Third Shift 4:30 PM–7:00 PM
Caregiver Samantha

4:30–5:00	Underwear change & check readings	Walk around to back room for change and to stretch legs.
5:00–5:30	Dinner	In kitchen
5:30–6:15	Walk	Walk off dinner.
6:30	Bedtime	As it stays light longer, move dinner to 5:30 and bedtime to 7:00

Remember when I said nothing can be taken for granted? Well, do not just assume they are bathing properly or at all. Think about a toddler and how they need to be assisted with water temperature, using soap and water and actually bathing and hitting those "neglected" spots. Details on the schedule are important if you have a caregiver coming into the home to care for your loved one. You can't assume they will know what you expect unless you have it written out for them.

In the earlier stages, my mom was secretly bathing my dad. That's right! She was protecting her man of 59 years from humiliation or possible embarrassment. They have always been committed to each other and looking out for each other's best interest. No need to stop now!

Dad needed help. He became unsure of how to put the whole bath experience together. I mean there's this washcloth that to him might look like a sock or small pillow case, a bar of soap or maybe a potato and then this dangerous waterfall with rapids at the bottom continuously flowing that he could hear and feel but not (clearly) see. Dad became afraid of the water and couldn't navigate all the components of washing himself. My mom put towels on the floor, drenched a washcloth in warm water from the sink and lathered him up really well. She then had him step into the shower to rinse off, even though he was still afraid of the water. He managed through his daily fear of that waterfall because he trusted that my mom would be with him and take care of him. I learned later on that because of his condition, he really wasn't seeing the water because it was clear. Just imagine hearing a steady heavy stream of rushing water but not being able to see it or know for sure what it was or where it was coming from. I'm a bit anxious just thinking about it like that.

Dad's trust in my mom, helped him navigate this difficult time. You must recognize how important relationships are for someone with dementia. Closeness, trust and commitment are everything! That is all they will be able to rely on with any certainty. Even when they don't know it, or can't express it, they will *feel* it instinctively.

The first stage of dementia is mild or early stage. This stage is where most of us on-lookers will notice smaller changes but won't recognize "suspicious" behavior. The sufferer may not recognize it either or maybe they are in a bit of denial. Simple forgetfulness like misplacing car keys, missing an appointment or forgetting someone's name is often associated with the normal aging process. It's often affectionately referred to as have a "senior moment". The instances of "senior moments" are becoming more frequent and noticeable during this phase but still not enough to signal major concern so being tested for dementia will go unchecked. At this stage you may have even said, "Let's just keep an eye on them."

At this stage, living alone and managing daily activities and responsibilities is often not a concern; although, if we had insight into it being more than a "senior moment", I would begin a care plan with the help of the sufferer right then. They could be very instrumental in planning out what they want and how they want to live. They could probably even write out what they want their daily schedule to look like and what should be included that will bring them joy and comfort. What if they could begin journaling so every detail was in black and white and we didn't have to guess? That would be the perfect scenario, but most aren't afforded that opportunity. By the time they accept something is terribly wrong, it is almost too late for them to manage outlining and coordinating their own care.

What was noticeable in my dad at this stage can only be recounted in retrospect. One instance was dad's driving. He loved to drive and we would go on long trips growing up. As adults, he would still drive if we decided to visit family together. We mostly had car pools because there were too many of us once we had our own families. Occasionally it would just be us girls with mom and dad. On this one occasion, my sisters and I were with our parents coming from Columbus, Ohio. A very close cousin was in the hospital and not doing too well so a visit was in order.

On the way back, dad pulled off of the highway for the extended bathroom break and snack run. Once we were loaded back into his SUV, he pulled right out in front of oncoming traffic as we were getting onto the highway. He never stopped to let the oncoming cars pass before crossing over the lanes to the on ramp. It was like he saw them but never "looked" and was just driving on auto pilot. We all screamed and he acted like nothing was wrong ... weird!

The second stage is the Moderate stage of dementia. This stage is an emotional one! You're discovering your mother, father, husband or wife has this disease called dementia (whether Alzheimer's, Vascular, Lewy Body, etc.). You might have heard about it before but never had to confront it yourself. Or maybe you've seen it in another family member and your mind immediately takes you to the worst possible experiences. It's not a good place to be in during the second stage but know you will get through it and begin to live in the abundance of life still being lived by your loved one.

During the Moderate stage, the sufferer's deficiencies become much more apparent and they are unable to hide symptoms from family and friends. There may be some personality changes or behaviors that are totally out of character. They may need assistance with food choices, preparation or reminders to eat and drink. They are probably skipping bath time so hygiene will become an issue. You may notice that their clothes do not match or maybe they have a winter sweater on in the summer time. They no longer know how to pay bills or even understand responsibility of bills, money, etc. My dad became obsessed with his wallet and having money in it so my mom and sister would fill his wallet with ones or fives and he would take it out, count it and put it right back. Those bills were washed so many times in his clothes or thrown out so they had to be replaced until he moved past that stage altogether.

This is where your care plan really begins to count, but how do you know what is really needed? Take one or two full days to observe your loved one in action to see where you need to start with your care. Plan to spend the night and just watch them from morning to bed and through the night. Remember that just because they can bathe today doesn't mean they can bathe tomorrow. This cruel disease can literally change one's abilities overnight. Take a look at what they do from the moment they rise in the morning. What are they eating? Are they eating? How do they prepare food? How do they navigate around the house or outside of the house? How's their driving? Everything is fair game during the observation period. You will be surprised and concerned at what you see.

Believe it or not, many of our family members are still driving during this phase. I'm using the term "driving" assuming they are in charge of a vehicle and can maneuver and control it. Even if their symptoms are just at the beginning stage of moderate, it is time to confiscate the keys. They are a danger to themselves and to others. Having that conversation with them is not going to be easy. You may have to remove the car from their home or hide the car keys. Dad would be looking for his car keys so we would just help him search knowing we had taken them. He would eventually move on to something else and it became easier to shift his focus. Enlist the help of their physician and blame it on the physician every time your family member brings it up (we did). Someone has to take the fall for this one so it might as well be them. Don't worry, the next ones on you!

This is also a good time to consider helping them transition to a healthier diet, if needed. There are many things that contribute to how well they will tolerate the changes that are happening. Food is a contributor. Try limiting or eliminating extra sugar, processed foods and other unhealthy choices. Incorporate more fruits and veggies, but don't withhold food that they like if they won't immediately take to these changes. It's important to keep them eating so they don't lose weight or feel deprived.

Meal planning is necessary to make sure meals aren't missed and the combinations are nutritiously appropriate. You'd be surprised that something as simple as a lunch choice of a turkey sandwich and chips could look different if my dad prepared lunch. It might just consist of slices of bread and maybe chips. What happened to the filling in the sandwich?! You can't predict how turkey slices will be viewed by him and what should happen with those slices. Part of your plan is to make sure nutritional meals are prepared and presented to them to eat. It's not enough to leave a plate in the refrigerator for them to heat up. They may never even go to the refrigerator or may forget how to use the microwave or stove.

In one of my support groups, a woman purchased a few frozen dinners to get her mom through the lunch hour when she wasn't there. Noticing that the dinners were still in the freezer, she asked her mom if she wouldn't mind heating up a frozen dinner for her in the microwave. Needless to say, she discovered her mom had forgotten how to use the microwave so could not heat the food. So what harm was that? It meant that her mom hadn't been eating during the day.

During this phase your loved one may also begin picking over their food. Dad's taste buds changed and he said food tasted like cardboard in his mouth. We learned if we added heavy or spicy seasoning, he could taste the food. Of course there is a balance because you don't want to add lots of salt and cause

other problems. There are an abundant of season-
ings that have strong aromas and flavors without
adding extra sodium. Experiment with those. For
us, we needed to make sure dad ate so until this
phase leveled out, we let him eat whatever he could
get down. Sugary foods were always a winner! Not
the best nutritionally but sometimes you have to do
what is necessary. Again, this didn't last forever and
he is a good healthy eater now.

Scheduled water breaks became a game changer
for us. Early on dad was in and out of the emergency
room with dehydration. We allowed him to hydrate
himself prior to being clued in that he was forgetting to drink water on his own. We began to moni-
tor his fluid intake and actually incorporated it into
his daily schedule. We offered him water at certain
intervals throughout the day to make sure he was
getting in enough fluids. Sounds like we are micro-
managing him right? Well, we are! That is exactly
what it takes to keep him safe, healthy and happy!

Mental disconnects are happening and that
is cause for concern with nutrition, safety and
their general well-being. These disconnects make it
unsafe to leave the sufferer alone or unsupervised.
They may still be functioning somewhat normal in
certain areas but what about the areas that aren't
functional anymore? It is hard to predict when or
where a deficiency will occur. Being prepared is the

only way to avoid a situation and even then, things can still happen.

So now you've bathed them or supervised to ensure they've done it properly. They've had a nutritious meal. What else is missing? Physical activity and outdoor time.

Your loved one needs to be kept mobile as long as possible. There will come a time when those brain circuits will no longer work to tell their muscles to lift their legs and move their feet. The brain controls everything, and as they decline, they may lose more and more of their independence.

When Dad is a bit under the weather, taking him out for a walk or, more likely, a wheel in his wheel-chair just gives him LIFE! He will begin to chatter, point out trucks or cars that he likes. He loves to hum when it's gettin' good to him!

As a part of his daily routine, he is escorted around the house to stretch his legs. He is a fall risk now so we always keep our hands on him and he uses a walker for support. Stability will become a problem for your loved one as well. Keep them safe. Dad stands in the kitchen after breakfast to shuffle through the mail. Afterwards, we take him outside in the morning and then again in the afternoon after another indoor stroll. Don't let the sun go down without letting them breathe in fresh air and take in some sunshine. There's healing power in fresh air and sunshine, as any medical professional will tell you.

Dad also loves to go for car rides. We will take him out to the mountains because they are pretty close and easy to get to. The ride brings him so much joy and gives him that boost of energy and excitement. Take them with you as much as you can. They are still a person wanting variety of activity and interaction with the public. They are not to be put away as if life is over. Life is just beginning! A different life, but life all the same.

What I've learned in this stage is that it is a very unpredictable period. One day, it appears he is normal and nothing is wrong and the next he can't form complete thoughts or sentences. What I learned is that dad needed constant reassurance. The hardest part in this phase was that he was going between past and present realities; as well as, reality and fantasy. It wasn't so hard because of the inconsistency in time or place but because *he* knew and would become so confused and questioned himself. He would begin to say something and then say, "I can't remember what I'm trying to say." Or just the look of utter confusion on his face as he sat silently trying desperately to understand in his own mind what was happening. When he would begin talking and couldn't go on, I'd say, "That's okay dad. I know what you mean." Or, "It's okay dad."

I believe we all caught on and to help him continue on with his thoughts or story he was telling, we would fill in the words he couldn't remember or the thought he couldn't express. I'm pretty sure we were and still are a crutch for him in this way but I'd do it all over again. It made it easier for him to communicate uninterrupted by his bouts of forgetfulness and also made for some interestingly exaggerated stories! We always had plenty of laughs together over the direction our conversations took.

I also learned that our schedule wasn't static. We needed to alter it and incorporate more support ... physical support. This is where the support team comes together. Dad needed help getting out of the bed in the mornings, in and out of chairs, walking and put to bed at night. Sometimes it can take two of us plus the caregiver if he isn't feeling well. Physical support is a must during this phase.

This final stage called Severe or Late Stage is just that. To me this only means that the level of care has changed but the care schedule is pretty solid by now. This is the time that requires you to give it your all! The main objective in this phase is to keep your family member or patient comfortable and happy. Don't lose sight of that. There is not a cure for this disease and by now, you will accept it. Don't forget that they are still living. I hear and read about the person no longer being "in there". That is just not true! This is the time to love them more and enjoy your time together and continue to make memories.

The final stage means your mother, father, husband, wife, patient, etc. need more one-on-one care and attention. They can no longer care for their physical needs. They may, in a lot of cases, become immobile. They need to be bathed and dressed. They need to either be fed or need help feeding themselves. They cannot live independently or be left alone ... ever! Verbal communication may have deteriorated to the point of either a few words or none at all. Most become incontinent and need adult diapers. They are dependent on you for their every need.

By now you have refined their schedules and have a really good rhythm going. You don't let them lay around in bed all day but get them up and bathed each and every day at the same time. You provide healthy meals, offer plenty of water, supplement foods to keep them eating and let them enjoy some indulgences. You take them out and let them still be social, getting fresh air and sunshine daily. You are rocking right along!

So what's the deal with the "Severe or Final Stage?" I'm not sure what you are expecting but you've already been doing what is needed since the "Moderate or Mid Stage." That's right! You've gotten good! Really good! I'm not saying it's easy, but you can probably call yourself a professional at this point. You aren't alarmed anymore with memory, speech or physical impairments. You adapt as these things change from day to day and keep going through your day. This way of life can go on for a very long time. It becomes our new normal and we're okay with that. Our love has never wavered. Our love has not dissipated. My dad gets more love, affection and attention than ever! He is not lacking in that area. Feelings is what doesn't go away. He still feels love and he gives love in the way that he can. He rubs my face, he holds my hand or he will even kiss my cheek when I offer it to him. He is still William Chatmon, my dad, my daddy.

CHAPTER FIVE

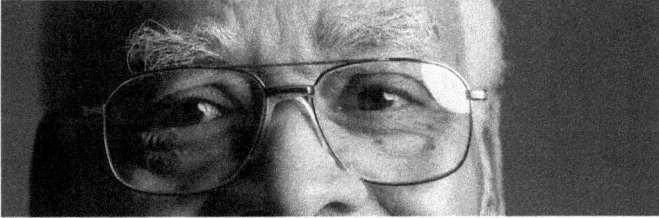

LIVE IN THE MOMENT — TOGETHER!

THIS IS THE FUN PART! I know you are still not there, but you'll get there. Trust me when I say it's not all doom and gloom. This is definitely an unexpected phase in life for your loved one and your family. You can choose to take it all in stride and adapt, or stay in the past and feel the heavy weight of depression and sadness all the time.

I remember the first time Dad's strange behavior seemed so uncharacteristic and disturbing. It was in the evening, and he was ready to go to bed. He went into his room to get ready for bed and came out in his underwear, undershirt, a belt around his waist and socks on his hands. At first we laughed. You know that nervous laugh – the one that comes out because you don't know what else to do? The Dad we knew *never* walked around in underwear! I might have seen him in his underwear once, maybe twice, in all of my years, and that was by total accident. So for him to just walk out – not just in his underwear but topped off with "accessories" – was just too heart-wrenching and painful to watch!

However, as we became more and more comfortable with odd behaviors or communication, we realized that, since he wasn't bothered by it, we shouldn't be either. He would say strange words, and we would all burst out laughing. If he thought what he said was funny and laughed uncontrollably, it was contagious, and we couldn't help but laugh too. We never laugh *at* him but *with* him. Now we can find humor in so many things, and we have a great time together.

I am *present* each day I am with him. What I mean by that is that I choose to live in the moment. If he needs help eating because he can't maneuver his fork, then I feed him. I don't put much thought into, "Oh, no! He can't feed himself today!" I don't overlook the changes, I'm not in denial about his condition and don't try to act like things haven't happened. I just choose to live with whatever the day brings and adapt to what his needs are.

You have to learn to accept the changes as quickly as you can wrap you mind around them. Sometimes it is hard to keep up, but acceptance is important in order to provide the necessary care.

Take your new relationship, new experiences and new-normal and embrace them. When others see your comfort level, it will help them get to where you are.

Now go! Live your life with your loved one! Start this new chapter by being educated, prepared, living in the moment and loving! In the end, love is all you need and all they want. That is the very thing they will not forget – how you make them feel every time you are around!

THE END OF *HIS* LETTER

Dad was diagnosed in the early spring of 2010. On December 9, 2010 my sister, Pam, presented a black leather bound journal to him because dad always loved to read, write and take lots of notes. Little did we know at that time, his reading and writing had started to deteriorate.

He began composing a letter to his family on December 27, 2010 and would only be able to complete three pages. It could be he had forgotten to continue writing because short-term memory was impaired or he couldn't keep his thoughts on track.

Nevertheless, there are only three full pages of his letter to us. Those three pages mean more to me than I can put into words. To still see his handwriting when now he can no longer write more than one random alphabet, warms my heart. It's almost funny how something as simple as a handwritten note can mean so much. It just makes me feel closer to him I guess.

Six years after he had begun composing this letter to us, I found his journal for the first time in a box where he kept lots of other important papers. He always kept our report cards from elementary school, certificates of birth from five children being born in different parts of the world, to immunizations that we all needed at some point in time.

At the time when dad began writing in this journal, he knew his memory was failing. In retrospect, he began writing at a time which seemed to us like a rapid explosion of dementia-like behaviors revealed themselves. I didn't know he was writing in his journal but when I stumbled across it and looked at the date, I realized he was trying to leave us with his life, his thoughts and I imagine words for the future. I am sad he couldn't finish our letter but feel comforted having these three full pages of his handwriting, his words, his feelings, and his thoughts. This is page one:

Dec 27, 2010

Dear Family,

I have been blessed to come to this day in my life full of joy & appreciation for my family. They are my greatest joy and happiness of my life

Let {me} say upfront that my greatest joy and appreciation is for my wife, Catherine. Anything that I have done or achieved she inspired. When I began my journey into manhood I never dreamed that I would meet and be able to claim a mate as beautiful, loving and talented as Catherine.

"Cathy", my short name for her was, is and always has been the tornado in my life. She is the greatest wife, mother, lover and friend. Cathy {never} met a challenge she didn't overcome.

*Note: before I continue you need to know that I began my journey in the cotton/tobacco {fields} of North Carolina on December 9, 1934.

Dec 27, 2010

Dear Family,
I have been Blessed To Come To This
day in my Life Full of Joy & Appreciation For
my Family. They Are My Greatest Joy And
Happiness of my Life
    Let say up front That My Greatest Joy
and Appreciation is For my Wife
CATHERINE. Any Thing That I have done
or Achieved She INSPIRED. When I
began my Journey into Manhood I Never
dreamed that I Would Meet And Able To
Claim A Mate As beautiful, Loving And
Talented As CATHERINE.
    "CATHY, my Short Name For Her, Was,
is And Always has been A TORNADO in
my Life", She is The Greatest
Wife, Mother, Lover And Friend." CAThy
Met A challenge She didnt overcome.

Growing 9 to 18 years of age as a youngster doing farm labor with a dream of wanting to become a soldier. I kept that dream to myself until 17 years of age where I informed my mother of my dream. She was not shocked but encouraged me to follow my dream.

I enlisted in the Air Force at the tender age of 18 and my life was changed forever. It took me many years to understand that life is a long and blessed journey. There were many starts, stops, delays, disappointments, but mostly joys over the lst 58 years. I still believe that country life should be experienced by all young males. It provides a greater appreciation of what is to come.

I began by raising my right

Growing to 18 years of age as a youngster doing FARM Labor with a dream of wanting to become a soldier. I kept that dream to my self until 17 years of age where I informed my mother of my dream. She was not shocked, but encouraged me to follow my dream.

I Enlisted in the Airforce at the Tender Age of 18, and my life was changed forever. It took me many years to understand that life is a long and blessed journey. There were many starts, stops, delays, ~~disappoint~~ dissapointments, but mostly joys over the last 58 years.

I still believe that country life should be experienced by all young males. It provides a greater appreciation of what is to come.

I began by raising my right

Hand and swearing alligence to my country by serving in the United States Air Force, April 3, 1953, and getting on an air plane (fear) for San Antonio Texas for basic training There were many starts & stops over the years. Smokey Hill Air Force base, Salina Kanses, June 1953 – May 1954, West Drayton England June 1954 – 1957, Lock Bourne Air Force Base Columbus, Ohio 1957 – September – September 1958

Pause = Where I met and married the woman of my dreams "Catherine Warren" and my life has never been the same. I will explain later:

I was reassigned (we were) reassigned to Chateaufoux Fra{n}ce in September of 1958 for 3 years where we gave birth to our oldest daugher Pamela Elaine, and oldest son, Will Thomas Jr. We had a great 3 year vacation there and got paid to enjoy ourselves. That tour provided great educational experiences and the joy of discovery in France.

Hand and Swearing Alligence to
My Country by Serving in The
United States Air Force, April 3, 1953,
and Getting on an Air plane (FEAR)
for San Antonio Texas For Basic Training
There were many starts & stops over
the years. Smokey Hill Air force Base Salina
Kanses, June 1953 - May 1954, West Drayton England
June 1954 - 1957, Lockbourne Air Force Base
Columbus, Ohio 1957 - September to September
1958. Pause - Where I met and married
the woman of my Dreams "Catherine Warren"
and my life Has Never Been the same.
I will explain later.
I was Reassigned (We were) Reassigned
to Chateauroux France in September of
1968 for 3 years where we gave Birth
to our oldest Daughter Pamela Elaine,
and oldest son, William Thomas JR.
We had a Great 3 year Vacation
there and Got Paid to Enjoy
ourselves. That Town provided
Great Educational Experiences and
The Joy of Discovery in France.

Knowing my dad, his values and what was important to him (God and family), I'm going to end his letter the way I imagine he would have if he could have.

... Family, I've given you all that I have. I've taught you to live a good, honest and productive life. I've taught you to stand up for what you believe in. I've taught you to always hold your head up high not to be arrogant but confident in who you are. I've shown you through my actions to provide for your family and to also do for others. I've taught you the importance of keeping each other close. Most importantly, I've taught you to pray, love God and put His will first in your lives. I want you to know how deeply I care and love each one of you and your uniqueness.

Pam, I know you are the oldest and are still bossing everyone around. You took up my passion for cooking for the family. Continue to prepare all the family meals because that is what keeps us together and happy. This is how I showed my love for you guys and now you are showing that same love in the same way. I have enjoyed your meals and the care that you show us with each plate prepared for me. I know you will always make sure I am well fed and for that I say, Thank You!

Tommy, as my oldest son, you will be responsible for making sure everyone stays in line and together. You will be that ear that each of your siblings will come to in my stead. Show them the love and compassion that you have within you. I also notice you are becoming more involved in assisting me as I need it. I want you to know that I would not be able to walk this road without you taking the reins and I thank-you for it.

Melodie, God gifted you with a voice that soothes the broken-hearted and moves us all to tears. Keep singing to me and to others. I will remember your voice when I hear it and it will bring me such comfort and joy.

Shelley, you were always the quieter one of the bunch. Somehow you broke free and became out-spoken in pursuit of your dreams. Continue to use your gifts to push through any barriers and over any boundaries. You are a fire cracker just like your mother (I didn't see that coming)! And, yes I still think you should work on that Doctorate degree.

Kevin, you're like me in so many ways. Large in stature, quiet in tone and strong in resolve. Don't be afraid to show your love and tender side too. You're a hard worker as I was but it's okay to slow down, relax a bit and just enjoy your family. At the end of the day, your family is your everything.

Tommy and Kevin, take care of my wife, your mother. I'm entrusting her to you and you know I will "bust some heads" over her!

I had to save the best for last. My wife, Hun, Cathy, Cath, the love of my life, the "Tornado in my life", my everything, you mean the world to me. We've prayed together, raised our children together, traveled together and stuck together for almost 60 years (so far). I expect to be reunited with you in heaven but until then your name and face will forever be etched in my mind and on my heart. Even if I can't say the words or understand the meanings of words, I will always look at you and know who you are...my wife, my love, my life!

I'm leaving you with this charge. My wife, my children and grandchildren, I want to see you in heaven. I want to see every one of my family there! I want to tell you that I know how well you took care of me and how much loved I felt during this trial. Don't disappoint me... I need to see you there.

Until we meet again!

Forever your dad and to Cathy, your husband,

I Love you all always!

Appendix

Video & Online Resources
Website – www. dadsgotdementia.com
Facebook (Vlog)-Dad's got Dementia
www.facebook.com/dadsgotdementia

To book Shelley Hall
email us at: info@dadsgotdementia.com

About the Author

SHELLEY CHATMON HALL, author of *Dad's got Dementia — Life after Diagnosis*, through the care of her father, has become a go-to expert resource for tips on everyday care. She is an accomplished vlogger and a sought after presenter who provides a wealth of practical information that most families can readily adopt when supporting a loved one dealing with this disease. To contact Shelley, please visit ***www.dadsgotdementia.com***

www.ingramcontent.com/pod-product-compliance
Lightning Source LLC
Chambersburg PA
CBHW071340290326
41933CB00040B/1825